Table of contents

Foreword

This book aims to provide a library of intelligent and highly accessible books - written by specialists in their various fields - for people who may not want to afford psychotherapy. This book is designed to provide readers with easily applicable techniques to help improve health and recovery from the condition discussed. The book discussed all aspects of a healthy life. Living a stress-free life is not something to be taken lightly.

INTRODUCTION

The start of a new decade brings with it new resolutions to improve one's life, including adopting a healthier lifestyle. In this book, you will learn more practical health tips that will make it easier for you to start living a healthy life.

Small changes can add up to big health benefits. We all have those well-meaning moments when we decide to make a fundamental change in our lifestyle: quitting smoking. Lose 20 lbs. Join a gym and start exercising every day.
While we should always strive to achieve these types of health goals, the journey to better health doesn't always have to involve big leaps. There are also many smaller steps you can take to improve your overall health and quality of life – and because these are things you can easily incorporate into your routine; They are easy to maintain in the long term. Even if you only have a few minutes, you can use that time to increase your well-being.

Health Rules

Healthy Eating

Eat a combination of different foods, including fruits, vegetables, legumes, nuts, and whole grains. Adults should eat at least five servings (400 g) of fruits and vegetables a day. You can improve your fruit and vegetable intake by always including vegetables in your meals; eat fresh fruits and vegetables as a snack; eat a variety of fruits and vegetables; and eat them in season. By eating healthy, you reduce the risk of malnutrition and non-communicable diseases (NCDs) such as diabetes, heart disease, stroke and cancer.

Use Less Salt And Sugar

Filipinos consume twice the recommended amount of sodium, which puts them at risk for hypertension, which in turn increases their risk of heart disease and stroke. Most people get sodium through salt. Reduce your salt intake to 5g per day, which equates to about a teaspoon. This is easier to do by limiting the amount of salt, soy sauce, fish sauce, and other sodium-rich spices when preparing

meals; remove salt, herbs and spices from your table; avoiding salty snacks; and choosing low sodium products.

On the other hand, consuming excessive amounts of sugar increases the risk of tooth decay and unhealthy weight gain. In both adults and children, free sugar intake should be reduced to less than 10% of total energy intake. This equates to 50g or about 12 teaspoons for an adult. The WHO recommends consuming less than 5% of total energy intake for additional health benefits. You can reduce your sugar intake by limiting your intake of sugary

snacks, sweets, and sugary drinks.

Reduce your intake of harmful fats

Fats consumed should represent less than 30% of your total energy intake.

This helps prevent unhealthy weight gain and non-communicable diseases. There are different types of fats, but unsaturated fats are preferred over saturated fats and trans fats. WHO recommends reducing saturated fats to less than 10% of total energy intake; reduce trans fats to less than 1% of total energy intake; and replacing both saturated and
trans fats with unsaturated ones.
The preferred unsaturated fats are found in fish, avocado and walnuts and in sunflower, soy, rapeseed and olive oils; saturated fats are found in fatty meats, butter, palm and coconut oil, cream, cheese, clarified butter and lard; and trans fats are found in baked and fried foods and in snacks and prepackaged foods, such as frozen pizzas, cookies, biscuits and cooking oil and spreads.

Avoid the harmful use of alcohol

There is no safe level for drinking

alcohol. Alcohol consumption can lead to health problems such as mental and behavioral disorders, including alcohol addiction, serious non-communicable diseases such as liver cirrhosis, certain cancers and heart disease, as well as injuries from violence and collisions and collisions on the road.

Don't smoke

Tobacco smoke causes non-communicable diseases such as lung disease, heart disease, and stroke. Tobacco kills not only direct smokers, but also non-smokers through second-hand exposure. Currently, there are approximately 15.9 million Filipino adults who smoke tobacco, but 7 out of 10 smokers are interested or intend to quit.
If you currently smoke, it's not too late to quit. Once you do this, you will experience immediate and long term health benefits.
If you're not a smoker, that's great! Don't start smoking and fight for your right to breathe tobacco-free air.

Be active

Physical activity is defined as any movement of the body produced by skeletal muscles that consume energy. This includes exercises and activities undertaken during work, play, housework, travel and recreation. The amount of exercise you need will depend on your age group, but adults between the ages of 18 and 64 should engage in at least 150 minutes of moderate-intensity physical activity during the week. Increase moderate-intensity physical activity to 300 minutes per week for additional health benefits.

Check your blood pressure regularly

Hypertension, or hypertension, has been called a "silent killer". This is because many people with hypertension may not be aware of the problem as they may have no symptoms. Left unchecked, hypertension can lead to heart, brain, kidney, and other diseases. Have your blood pressure checked regularly by a healthcare professional so that you know your numbers. If your blood pressure is high, ask a health professional for advice. This is crucial in preventing and managing hypertension.

Take the test

Getting tested is an important step in knowing your health, especially when it comes to HIV, hepatitis B, sexually transmitted diseases (STDs) and tuberculosis (TB). If left untreated, these diseases can lead to serious complications and even death. Knowing your status will help you know how to continue to prevent these illnesses or, if you are HIV-positive, get the care and treatment you need. Go to any public or private health facility, where you feel comfortable, to get tested.

Get vaccinated

Vaccination is one of the most effective measures to prevent the disease. Vaccines work with your body's natural defenses to boost protection against diseases such as cervical cancer, cholera, diphtheria, hepatitis B, influenza, measles, mumps, pneumonia, poliomyelitis, rabies, rubella, tetanus, typhoid and yellow fever.

In the Philippines, free vaccines are provided to children 1 year and under the Department of Health's routine immunization program. If you are a teenager or an adult, you can ask your doctor to check your vaccination status or if you want to get vaccinated.

Practice Safe Sex

Taking care of your sexual health is important for your overall health and well-being. Practice safer sex to prevent HIV and other sexually transmitted infections like gonorrhea and syphilis. There are preventative measures such as pre-exposure prophylaxis (PrEP) that protects you from HIV and condoms that protect you from HIV and other sexually transmitted diseases.

Cover your mouth when you cough or sneeze

Diseases such as the flu, pneumonia and tuberculosis are transmitted through the air. When an infected person coughs or sneezes, infectious agents can be transmitted to others through airborne droplets. If you experience coughing or sneezing, be sure to cover your mouth with a mask or use a tissue and then gently throw it away. If you don't have a tissue handy when you cough or sneeze, cover your mouth with the hollow (or inside) of your elbow as much as possible.

Prevent mosquito bites

Mosquitoes are one of the deadliest animals in the world. Diseases such as dengue fever, chikungunya, malaria and lymphatic filariasis are transmitted by mosquitoes and continue to afflict Filipinos. There are simple steps you can take to protect yourself and your loved ones from mosquito-borne diseases. If you're traveling to an area where mosquito-borne diseases are known, see a doctor for vaccinations to prevent illnesses such as Japanese encephalitis and yellow fever, or if you need to take antimalarial medication. Wear light-colored long-sleeved shirts and pants and use insect repellent. At home, use screens on windows and doors, use mosquito nets, and clean your surroundings weekly to destroy mosquito breeding grounds.

Obey traffic rules

Traffic accidents kill more than a million people

worldwide and injure millions more. Road acc idents can be prevented through various measures implemented by the government, such as: B. Strict legislation and enforcement, safer infrastructure and vehicle standards, and improved post-crash care. You can also prevent traffic accidents yourself by making sure you obey traffic rules, such as: For example, using the adult seat belt and child restraint system for your children, wearing a helmet when you drive a motorcycle or a bicycle, do not drink and drive and use yo ur mobile phone while driving.

Only drink clean water

Drinking unsafe water can lead to waterborne diseases such as cholera, diarrhea, hepatitis A, typhoid and poliomyelitis. At least 2 billion people worldwide use a drinking water source contaminated with faeces. Check with your water dealer and water filling station to make sure the water you drink is safe. In an environment where you are unsure of your water source, boil the water for at least one minute. This destroys the harmful organisms in the water. Let it cool naturally before drinking.

Breastfeed babies between the ages of 0 and 2

Breastfeeding is the best way to give babies and children the ideal nutrition. WHO advises mothers to start breastfeeding within one hour of giving birth? Breastfeeding for the first six months is crucial for healthy baby growth. It is recommended that breastfeeding continue for up to two years and beyond. Apart from being beneficial for babies, breastfeeding is also good for the mother as it reduces the risk of breast and ovarian cancer, type II diabetes and postpartum depression.

Talk to someone you trust when you feel down

Depression is a common disease worldwide with over 260 million people affected. Depression can manifest itself in a number of ways, but it can make you feel hopeless or worthless, or think a lot about negative and distressing thoughts, or feel a sense of overwhelming pain. If you are experiencing this, remember that you are not alone. Talk to someone you trust, such as a family member, friend, colleague, or mental health professional, about how you feel

Take antibiotics only as prescribed

Antibiotic resistance is one of the greatest threats to public health of our generation. When antibiotics lose their potency, bacterial infections become more difficult to treat, leading to higher medical costs, longer hospital stays and increased mortality. Antibiotics lose their potency due to improper and excessive use in humans and animals. Be sure to only take antibiotics when prescribed by a qualified doctor. And after the prescription, carry out the treatment days as indicated. Never share antibiotics.

Clean your hands well

Hand hygiene is essential not just for healthcare workers, but for everyone. Clean hands can prevent the spread of infectious diseases. You should wash your hands with soap and water if your hands are visibly dirty, or you should scrub them with an alcohol-based product.

Prepare food correctly

Dangerous foods containing harmful bacteria, viruses, parasites or chemicals cause more than 200 diseases ranging from diarrhea to cancer. When buying food at the market or store, check the actual labels or products to make sure it is safe to eat. When preparing food, be sure to follow the five keys to safer food: (1) stay clean; (2) separated raw and cooked; (3) cook thoroughly; (4) store food at safe temperatures; and (5) use safe water and resources.

Get regular checkups

Regular checkups can help detect health problems before they start. Healthcare professionals can help detect and diagnose health problems early when the options for treatment and cure are greatest. Visit the nearest health facility to view the health services, screenings and treatments available to you.

Ways You Can Improve Your Health

Small changes can add up to big health benefits. We all have those well-meaning moments when we decide to make a fundamental change in our lifestyle: quitting smoking. Lose 20 lbs. Join a gym and start exercising every day.

While we should always strive to achieve these types of health goals, the journey to better health doesn't always have to involve big leaps.

There are also many smaller steps you can take to improve your overall health and quality of life – and because these are things you can easily incorporate into your routine; They are easy to maintain in the long term. Even if you only have a few minutes, you can use that time to increase your well-being.

Try incorporating the following activities and strategies into your day. When these simple steps become habits, they can have a huge positive effect on your overall health.

Enjoy stress relief: Experts recommend

regular exercise, meditation, and breathing techniques to reduce stress. But something as simple — and enjoyable — as listening to soothing music, reading a good book, soaking in a hot tub, or playing with your pet can also help you relax.

Heed this advice, as prolonged stress can cause or worsen a number of health problems, including heart disease, stroke, high blood pressure, depression, ulcers, irritable bowel syndrome, migraines and obesity.

Don't have much time? Don't let that stress you out. As with exercise, short periods of relaxation are also beneficial.

Spending even 10 minutes at a time doing something you enjoy can go a long way in overcoming the stressors of everyday life. Just reading a chapter or taking your dog for a few laps around the block will make you feel calmer, cooler, and more energetic.

If you can't take a full break from what you're doing, just try taking a few slow, deep breaths at this time. Slowing down your breathing will help you relax. This relaxation response releases chemicals from the body that relieve stress and can improve immune function.

Deep breathing can also lower your resting heart rate. People with a lower resting heart rate are generally in better physical condition than people with a higher heart rate.

Get rid of the salt: A salt shaker on the dining table makes it all too easy to consume excess salt, which can lead to hypertension. Then put the shaker in a cupboard or pantry and only take it out when you are cooking.

It is also a good idea to sample the food before salting it. You may find that it doesn't need anything else.

You can also try flavoring your food with lemon or lime juice,
garlic, chili flakes, herbs, or a salt-free spice blend. Fill your fridge and pantry with your favorite fresh and dried herbs so you always have them on hand to flavor your food.

Go to bed first: Most of us can't sleep the seven or more hours that adults need.

Over time, a lack of closed eyes can increase the risk of heart attack or stroke, regardless of age, weight, or exercise habits.

If you're constantly sleep deprived, going to bed even 15 minutes
earlier each night can help. Plus, set and stick to a regular sleep and wake schedule, even on days off.

Drink a glass of red wine: Studies have shown that the powerful antioxidants in red wine protect against heart disease, colon cancer, anxiety and depression. So unless there's a medical reason you shouldn't be drinking, go ahead and enjoy that glass of merlot with your evening meal - you can even toast your good health.

Drink in moderation: Just as a small amount of red wine has health benefits, too much alcohol, even red wine, can cause various health problems, including liver and kidney disease and cancer.
Women in particular should be careful when drinking alcohol. They have a higher overall risk of liver problems than men, so they are more likely to have liver problems from small amounts of alcohol.
For a healthy man, two drinks a day probably won't hurt; Women, on the other hand, should limit themselves to one alcoholic drink a day.

Check your posture and ergonomics: Next time you're sitting at your desk or on the phone, take a moment to think about your posture. Next, straighten your back, tuck your stomach in, and place your feet flat on the floor with your legs uncrossed. You will immediately feel more relaxed. The few seconds it takes can help you avoid back pain, one of the most common health problems in the United States and a leading cause of disability.

And when working at a computer, pay attention to the ergonomics of your workspace, i.e. how you blend and move into your environment, to avoid back and neck pain. , carpal tunnel syndrome, eye strain and other work-related injuries.

A few simple adjustments, like repositioning your computer screen, switching to a chair that provides more lower back support, and taking regular breaks throughout the day to stretch, can go a long way toward creating a healthier and more comfortable workspace.

The next time you go up to a higher floor, bypass the elevator and go up the stairs instead. You get your blood pumping, you work your lungs, and you work your lower body muscles.

Create a crossword puzzle: Rush researchers found that mentally demanding activities, such as reading, crosswords or Sodoku and chess, can have a protective effect on the brain.

According to research studies, engaging the mind regularly can help reduce the risk of dementia associated with

Alzheimer's disease.
Don't like puzzles or games? Don't worry: there are other ways to keep your brain healthy. Eat with your non-dominant hand. Take a new route home from work. And network with others – social engagement can also protect against dementia.

Weight: Maintaining a healthy weight can reduce your risk of heart disease, stroke, and certain cancers. But for women, there's another reason to prevent weight gain: it will reduce the risk of future pelvic floor disorders.
Pelvic floor disorders are more common in women who have had a vaginal birth. However, a recent study found that even women who have never had a vaginal birth are at increased risk of stress urinary incontinence if they are overweight or obese.

Make some dietary substitutions:
• Replace white bread, rice, crackers, and pasta with healthier whole-grain versions.
• Use skinless chicken and turkey in your recipes instead of skinless, lean cuts of meat like beef or pork.
• Replace a sugary drink (soft drink, fruit juice, etc.) with a large glass of water

every day. • If you feel hungry between meals, instead of having candy bars or chips, snack on a handful of almonds or cashews, a piece of whole fruit, or carrot sticks dipped in hummus.

Also try to include an extra serving of non-starchy vegetables in your daily diet.

want a snack Eat a carrot instead of a cookie. Cooking dinner for your family? Instead of mashed potatoes, serve broccoli or spinach on the side. Add green peas to your brown rice or slices of red or yellow pepper to your sandwich.

It's no secret

that vegetables, especially dark leafy greens, ar e good for your health. But there's another benefit to including more vegetables in your daily diet: they're high in fiber and high in water, which helps you feel full and satisfied without too many calories and fat.

Take the stairs: The next time you go up to a higher floor, bypass the elevator and go up the stairs instead. You get your blood pumping, you work your lungs, and you work your lower body muscles.

It's a great way to add physical activity to your day without having to block out time for exercise. If you're aiming for the recommended 10,000 steps per day, climbing stairs counts toward that total. All of these small steps can contribute to a healthier you.

Stretch it out: Stretching your muscles regularly can help prevent injury, stay limber, and move freely with age. Before and after exercise, take a few minutes to stretch. If you're not exercising that day, take a few breaks to stretch. Find a quiet place in the office where you won't be disturbed. On my way? Look for natural opportunities to stretch in your daily routine, such as B. getting out of the car or looking for items on a high shelf in the store.
Stretching right before bed can also help you release tension and help you fall asleep. And balance exercises — like tai chi — can help significantly reduce the risk of dangerous falls.

Look ahead

The good news is that it is never too early, nor too late, to adopt healthy habits. When you are young, you can lay the foundation for a healthy life. As you get older, healthy habits can help you manage any diseases you may have and reduce your risk of contracting other diseases in the future.

Healthy Eating Tips

1. Choose good carbs, not no carbs.
Whole grain products are the best choice.
2. Pay attention to the protein packet. Fish, poultry, nuts and beans are the best choices.
3. Choose foods with healthy fats, limit foods high in saturated fats and avoid foods with trans fats. Vegetable oils, nuts and fish are the healthiest sources.
4. Eat a fiber-rich diet rich in whole grains, vegetables, and fruits.
5. Eat more vegetables and fruits. Go for color and variety - dark green, yellow, orange and red.
6. Calcium is important. But milk is not the only or even the best source.
7. Water is the best way to quench your thirst. Avoid sugary drinks and save milk and juice. 8. Eating less salt is good for everyone's health. Choose more fresh foods and less processed foods.
9. Moderate alcohol consumption can be healthy, but not for everyone. You have to weigh the benefits and risks.
10. A daily multivitamin is excellent nutritional insurance. A little extra vitamin D can give your health an extra boost.

Health and nutrition advice

It's easy to get lost when it comes to health and nutrition. Even qualified experts often seem to have conflicting opinions, which can make it hard to figure out what you should actually be doing to optimize your health. But despite all the disagreements, some wellness tips are well backed by research.

Limit sugary drinks

Sugary drinks like sodas, fruit juices and sweetened teas are the main sources of added sugar in the American diet.

Unfortunately, the results of several studies suggest that sugary drinks increase the risk of heart disease and type 2 diabetes, even in people who do not have excess body fat.

Sugary drinks are also particularly harmful to children, as they can contribute not only to childhood obesity, but also to conditions that typically don't develop until adulthood, such as type 2 diabetes, high blood pressure and non-alcoholic fatty liver disease.

Healthier alternatives include:
- Water
- unsweetened teas
- Sparkling water
- Coffee

Eat nuts and seeds

Some people avoid nuts because they are high in fat. However, nuts and seeds are incredibly nutritious. They are rich in protein, fiber and a variety of vitamins and minerals.
Walnuts can help you lose weight and reduce the risk of developing type 2 diabetes and heart disease.
Additionally, a large observational study found that low intake of nuts and seeds may have been linked to an increased risk of death from heart disease, stroke, or type 2 diabetes.

Avoid ultra-processed foods

Ultra-processed foods are foods that contain ingredients that have been significantly altered from their original form. They often contain additives such as added sugar, highly refined oil, salt,

preservatives, artificial
sweeteners, colors and flavors.

Examples include:

- Little cake
- Fast food
- Frozen food
- Canned products
- Chips

Highly processed foods
are very palatable, which means they are easily over-consumed and
activate reward regions in the brain, which can lead to excessive calorie expenditure and weight gain. Studies show that a diet high in ultra-processed foods can contribute to obesity, type 2 diabetes, heart disease and other chronic diseases.
Along with low-quality ingredients
like flammable fats, added sugars, and refined grains, they're generally low in fiber, protein, and micronutrients. So they usually provide empty calories.

Don't be afraid of coffee

Despite some controversy over this, coffee
is packed with health benefits.

It's packed with antioxidants, and some studies have linked coffee intake to longevity and reduced risk of type 2 diabetes, Parkinson's and Alzheimer's, and a host of other diseases.
The most beneficial intake appears to be 3-4 cups a day, although pregnant people should limit or avoid it entirely as it has been associated with low birth weight.
However, it is best to consume coffee and all caffeine-based products in moderation.
Excessive caffeine intake can lead to health problems such as insomnia and heart palpitations. To enjoy coffee safely and healthily, limit your intake to less than 4 cups a day and avoid high-calorie, high-sugar additives like sweet cream.

Eat fatty fish

Fish is an excellent source of high quality protein and healthy fats. This is especially true for fatty fish like salmon, which are packed with anti-inflammatory omega-3 fatty acids and various other nutrients.
Studies show that people who regularly eat fish have a lower risk of various diseases, including heart

disease, dementia and inflammatory bowel disease.

Get enough sleep

The importance of getting enough quality sleep cannot be overstated.
Poor sleep can promote insulin resistance, disrupt your appetite hormones, and affect your physical and mental performance. In addition, lack of sleep is one of the most important individual risk factors for weight gain and obesity. People who don't get enough sleep tend to choose foods that are high in fat, sugar, and calories, which can lead to unwanted weight gain.

Feed your gut bacteria

The bacteria in your gut, known collectively as the gut microbiota, are extremely important for overall health. Disruption of gut bacteria is linked to certain chronic diseases, including obesity and various digestive problems. Good ways to improve gut health include eating probiotic foods like yogurt and sauerkraut, taking probiotic supplements - when indicated - and eating plenty of fiber. Specifically, fiber serves as a prebiotic or food source for gut bacteria.

Stay hydrated

Hydration is an important and often overlooked indicator of health. Staying hydrated helps ensure that your body is functioning optimally and that your blood volume is adequate. Drinking water is the best way to stay hydrated because it's free of calories, sugar, and additives.

Although there is no set amount that everyone needs per day, try to drink enough to quench your thirst.

Don't eat heavily charred meat

Meat can be a nutritious and healthy part of your diet. It is very high in protein and a rich source of nutrients.

However, problems arise when the meat is charred or burnt. This charring can lead to the formation of harmful compounds that can increase your risk of certain types of cancer.

When cooking meat, try not to char or burn it. Also limit your intake of red and processed meats, such as deli meats and bacon, as they are linked to overall cancer risk and colon cancer risk.

Avoid bright lights before going to bed

When you are exposed to bright lights, which contain wavelengths of blue light, at night, it can interfere with the production of the sleep hormone melatonin.

Some ways to reduce blue light exposure are to wear blue light blocking glasses, especially if you have been using a computer or other digital display for a long time, and avoid digital displays 30 minutes to an hour before use.

This can help your body produce melatonin naturally at night, helping you sleep better.

Take vitamin D if you are deficient

Most people do not get enough vitamin D. While these widespread vitamin D deficiencies are not immediately harmful, maintaining adequate levels of vitamin D can help optimize health by improving bone strength, reducing symptoms of depression, strengthening the immune system and reducing the risk of cancer.

If you don't spend a lot of time in the sun, your vitamin D levels may be low.

If you have access, it's a good idea to have your levels tested so that you can correct your levels by supplementing with vitamin D if needed.

Eat lots of fruits and vegetables

Vegetables and fruits are packed with prebiotic fiber, vitamins, minerals and antioxidants, many of which have powerful health effects.

Studies show that people who eat more vegetables and fruits tend to live longer and have a lower risk of heart disease, obesity and other diseases.

Eat enough protein

Eating enough protein is essential for optimal health because it provides the raw materials your body needs to form new cells and tissues.

In addition, this nutrient is particularly important for maintaining a moderate body weight. A high protein intake can boost your metabolism - or burn calories - while making you feel full. It can also reduce cravings and your desire for a late night snack.

Get moving

Aerobic exercise, or cardio, is one of the best things you can do for your mental and physical health.

It is particularly effective in reducing belly fat, the harmful type of fat that accumulates around the organs. Reducing belly fat can lead to major improvements in metabolic health.

According to the physical activity guidelines for Americans, we should aim for at least 150 minutes of moderate-intensity activity per week.

Do not smoke or use drugs and only drink in moderation

Smoking, harmful drug use, and alcohol abuse can have serious negative health effects.

If you take any of these actions, consider reducing or quitting to reduce the risk of chronic disease. There are resources available online - and probably in your local community - to help you. Talk to your doctor to learn more about accessing resources.

Use extra virgin olive oil

Extra virgin olive oil is one of the healthiest vegetable oils you can use. It's packed with heart-healthy monounsaturated fats and powerful antioxidants with anti-inflammatory properties. Extra virgin olive oil may benefit heart health, as some evidence suggests that people who consume it have a reduced risk of dying from heart attacks and strokes.

Minimize your sugar intake

Added sugar is common in modern foods and beverages. High intake has been linked to obesity, type 2 diabetes and heart disease.

The Dietary Guidelines for Americans recommend keeping added sugar intake to less than 10% of your daily calorie intake, while the World Health Organization recommends reducing added sugars to 5% or less of your calorie intake. daily for optimal health.

Limit refined carbohydrate.

Not all carbohydrates are created equal. Refined carbohydrates are highly processed to remove their fiber. They are relatively poor in nutrients and can harm your health if consumed in excess. Most ultra-processed foods are made up of refined carbohydrates, such as processed corn, white flour, and added sugars. Studies show that a diet high in refined carbohydrates may be linked to overeating, weight gain, and chronic diseases such as type 2 diabetes and heart disease.

Lift heavy weights

Strength and resistance training is one of the best exercises you can do to build muscle and improve your body composition.

It can also lead to significant improvements in metabolic health, including better insulin sensitivity – which means your blood sugar is easier to control – and an increase in your metabolic rate, or the number of calories you burn at rest.

If you don't have weights, you can use your own body weight or resistance bands to build resistance and get a comparable workout with many of the same benefits

Avoid artificial trans fats

Artificial trans fats are harmful man-made fats that have been strongly linked to inflammation and heart disease.

Avoiding them should be a lot easier now that they've been banned in the US and many other countries altogether. Note that you may still come across certain foods that contain small amounts of natural trans fats, but these are not associated with the same negative effects as artificial trans fats.

Use lots of herbs and spices

Today more than ever we have a variety of herbs and spices available. Not only do they provide flavor, but they can also provide various health benefits.

For example, ginger and turmeric both have powerful anti-inflammatory and antioxidant effects, which can help improve your overall health.

Due to their powerful potential health benefits, you should aim to include a wide variety of herbs and spices in your diet.

Cultivate your social relationships

Social relationships - with friends, family and loved ones you care about - are important not only for your mental well-being, but also for your physical health.

Studies show that people who have close friends and family are healthier and live much longer than those who don't.

Track your food intake from time to time

The only way to know exactly how many calories you are consuming is to weigh your food and use a nutrition tracker, as estimating your portion sizes and calorie intake are unreliable.

Tracking can also provide information about your protein, fiber and micronutrient intake.

Although some studies have found a link between calorie tracking and disordered eating habits, there is evidence that people who track their food intake tend to be more successful at losing and maintaining weight.

Get rid of excess belly fat

Excess abdominal fat, or visceral fat, is a particularly harmful mode of fat distribution that is linked to an increased risk of cardiometabolic diseases such as type 2 diabetes and heart disease.

For this reason, your waist circumference and waist-to-hip ratio can be much stronger indicators of health than your weight. Cutting out refined carbs, eating more protein and fiber, and reducing stress (which can lower cortisol, a stress hormone that triggers belly fat deposition) are all strategies that can help you lose belly fat.

Avoid restrictive diets

Diets are generally ineffective and rarely work well in the long term. In fact, a past diet is one of the strongest predictors of future weight gain.

This is because overly restrictive diets reduce your metabolism or the amount of calories you burn, making weight loss more difficult. At the same time, they also

cause changes in hunger and satiety hormones, making you hungrier and can trigger a craving for foods high in fat, calories and sugar.
All of this is a recipe for rebound weight gain, or "yo-yo" diet.
Instead of dieting, try to adopt a healthier lifestyle. Focus on feeding your body instead of depriving it.
Weight loss should follow as you switch to whole, nutritious foods, which are naturally more filling and lower in calories than processed foods.

Eat whole eggs

Despite the constant back and forth about eggs and health, it is a myth that eggs are unhealthy due to their cholesterol content. Studies show they have minimal effects on blood cholesterol levels in the majority of people and are an excellent source of protein and nutrients. Additionally, a review of 263,938 people found that egg intake was not associated with cardiovascular disease risk.

Meditate

Stress has a negative effect on your health. It

can affect blood sugar, food choices, disease susceptibility, weight, fat distribution, and more. For this reason, it is important to find healthy ways to manage stress. Meditation is one such pathway, and there is scientific evidence supporting its use to manage stress and improve health.

In a study of 48 people with high blood pressure, type 2 diabetes, or both, researchers found that meditation helped reduce LDL (bad) cholesterol and inflammation compared to the control group. In addition, participants in the meditation group reported an improvement in their mental and physical well-being.

The final result

A few simple steps can go a long way towards improving your eating habits and your well-being.

However, if you're trying to live a healthier life, don't just focus on the foods you eat. Exercise, sleep and social relationships are also important.

With the evidence-based tips above, it's easy to make small changes that can have a big impact on your overall health.

Try it today: This list has many suggestions that can help improve your health, but it's best to practice only one or two at a time so you don't burn out. The more these healthy actions become habits, the more you can add to your routine.

Simple Rules For Incredible Health

Following a healthy lifestyle often seems incredibly complicated. Advertisements and experts around you seem to be giving conflicting advice.

However, living a healthy life doesn't have to be complicated.

To achieve optimal health, lose weight and feel better every day, all you need to do is follow these simple rules.

Do not introduce toxic substances into your body

A lot of things people put in their bodies are downright toxic. Some, such as cigarettes, alcohol, and narcotics, are also highly addictive, making it difficult for people to abandon or avoid them.

If you have a problem with any of these substances, diet and exercise are the least of your worries.

While alcohol in moderation is good for those who can tolerate it, tobacco and drugs are bad for everyone.

But an even more common problem today is

eating unhealthy, disease-promoting junk food.

If you want to achieve optimal health, you should minimize your consumption of these foods. Probably the most effective change you can make to improve your diet is to cut down on processed and packaged foods. This can be difficult, as many of these foods are designed to be extremely palatable and difficult to resist.

When it comes to specific ingredients, added sugars are among the worst. These include sucrose and high fructose corn syrup.

Both can wreak havoc on the metabolism when consumed in excess, although some people can tolerate moderate amounts. Also, it's a good idea to avoid all trans fats, which are found in some types of margarine and packaged baked goods.

SUMMARY

You cannot be healthy if you continue to inject disease-promoting substances into your body. This includes tobacco and alcohol, but also some processed foods and ingredients.

Lift objects and move

Using your muscles is extremely important for

optimal health. While weight lifting and exercise can definitely help you look better, improving your appearance is just the tip of the iceberg.
You also need to exercise to keep your body, brain and hormones functioning optimally. Lifting weights lowers blood sugar and insulin levels, improves cholesterol, and lowers triglycerides.
It also increases testosterone and growth hormone levels, both of which are associated with better well-being.

Additionally, exercise can help reduce depression and the risk of several chronic diseases, such as obesity, type 2 diabetes, heart disease, Alzheimer's disease, and many others.
Additionally, exercise can help you lose fat, especially when combined with a healthy diet. It not only burns calories but also improves hormone levels and overall body function.
Fortunately, there are many ways to exercise. You don't have to go to the gym or own expensive exercise equipment. You can practice for free and in the comfort of your own home. Just search Google or YouTube for things like "bodyweight workouts" or "calisthenics".
Going out for a walk or a walk is another

important thing to do, especially if you can get some sun while you're at it (for a natural source of vitamin D). Walking is a great choice and a highly underrated form of exercise.
The key is to pick something you like and can stick with for the long term. If you are out of shape or have a medical condition, it is a good idea to talk to your doctor or a
qualified healthcare professional before starting any new fitness program. exercises.

SUMMARY
Not only does exercise make you look better, but it also improves your hormone levels, makes you feel better, and lowers your risk of various diseases.

Sleep like a baby

Sleep is very important for overall health, and studies show that sleep deprivation is correlated with many illnesses, including obesity and heart disease.
It is strongly recommended that you take the time to get a good quality night's sleep.
If you feel like you're not sleeping well, there are several ways you can try to improve it:

- Don't drink coffee at the end of the day.

• Try to go to bed and wake up at the same time every day.
• Sleeping in complete darkness, without artificial lighting.
• Turn down the lights in the house a few hours before going to bed.
• Refer to this article for more tips on how to improve sleep. It may also be a good idea to consult your doctor. Sleep disorders such as sleep apnea are common and in many cases easily treatable.

SUMMARY
Good sleep can improve your health in more ways than you can imagine. You will feel better physically and mentally, which will reduce your risk of various health problems.

Avoid excessive stress

A healthy
lifestyle includes a healthy diet, good sleep, and regular exercise.
But how you feel and how you think is also very important. Being stressed out all the time is a recipe for disaster.
Excessive stress can raise cortisol levels and

severely damage your metabolism. It can increase cravings
for junk food, stomach fat, and the risk of various diseases. Studies also show that stress is a major contributing factor to depression, which is a huge health problem today.
To reduce stress, try to make your
life easier: exercise, take nature walks, practice deep breathing techniques, and maybe even meditation.
If you absolutely can't handle the burdens of your daily life without being overly stressed, consider consulting a psychologist.
Overcoming stress will not only make you healthier, it will also improve your life in other ways. Going through life worried, anxious and never being able to relax and have fun is a big waste.

SUMMARY
Stress can wreak havoc on your health, leading to weight gain and
various illnesses. There are many
ways to reduce your stress.

Feed your body real food

The easiest and most effective way to eat

healthy is to focus on real foods.

Choose whole, unprocessed foods that resemble what they look like in nature. It is best to eat a combination of animals and plants: meat, fish, eggs, vegetables, fruits, nuts, seeds, as well as healthy fats, oils and high-fat dairy products.

If you are healthy, lean, and active, eating whole, unrefined carbohydrates is absolutely fine. These include potatoes, sweet potatoes, legumes, and whole grains such as oats.

However, if you are overweight or obese or have shown signs of metabolic problems such as diabetes or metabolic syndrome, cutting down on your major carbohydrate sources can lead to dramatic improvements. People can often lose a lot of weight simply by cutting down on carbohydrates because they subconsciously start eating less. Whatever you do, try to choose whole, unprocessed foods rather than foods that look like they were made in a factory.

SUMMARY

Choosing whole, unprocessed foods like fruits, vegetables, seeds, and whole grains is very important for your health.

You have to stick to it for life

It's important to keep in mind that a dieting mindset is a bad idea because it almost never works in the long run.
For this reason, it is important to aim for a lifestyle change.
Being healthy is a marathon, not a sprint.
It takes time and you have to do it for the rest of your life.
'Slow but steady' wins the slimming contest

People whose weight fluctuates at the start of a weight loss program have worse long-term results.

If losing weight feels more like a yo-yo than a ball rolling down a rolling hill, you may want to rethink your approach.
A new study found that people whose weight fluctuated in the first few months of a weight loss program lost less weight over the long term than people who made more consistent progress week after week.
Researchers at Drexel
University have suggested that this could help identify people who need additional early-stage support to achieve their weight loss goals. The dangers of

regaining lost weight are nothing new to medical professionals.

If you're yo-yo, that's a clear sign or red flag that it's about more than the food you eat and the exercise you do, that there are probably ingrained behavioral patterns that we need to watch to change to be sure. ensure long-term membership, which was not involved in the study.

Yo-yo diets lead to less success

People whose weight fluctuated more in the first 6 or 12 months lost less weight after one and two years.

For example, people who lost four pounds in one week, gained two the next, and lost another pound the next, fared worse than people who lost one pound each week for the first six months.

While weight variability in the first six months predicted long-term success, the researchers found that the 12-month variability was less affected by other factors.

All volunteers were given goals to focus on during the program, such as monitoring their habits, progress and calorie intake, while also increasing their physical activity. The first six months of the program focused on weight loss, with weekly sessions in small groups. The last six months have gone into weight maintenance, with less frequent sessions.

People who reported more binge eating, emotional eating, and food concern at the start of the study showed greater weight variability and lost less weight after a year or two.

This suggests that weight variability is a better predictor of long-term success than one's relationship to food.

Weight variability causes poorer weight loss outcomes. But it can help target people who don't benefit from a particular weight loss program, before trying to lose weight for a year.

While losing 10 pounds in the first week can be a big motivator for many people, in the long run it might not matter if your weight is on the rise the rest of the time.

Over the course of the 30-week show, people lost an average of 129 pounds each. But six years later, all but one had regained most of their weight, an average of 90 pounds each.

Develop sustainable weight loss

Doing things like severely limiting calories or ditching carbohydrates can give you dramatic weight loss results - they're not helpful if you want lifelong success. The types of long-term sustainable behavioral changes. Of course, these don't lead to as sexy results as losing 10 pounds in a week.

Sexy or not, sustainable is fine if you want to maintain your weight.

One way to sustainably address weight loss is to set goals that you can actually achieve.

For example, if your approach to weight loss involves running and you currently run a mile three times a week, the next step should be doable. That could mean running 2 miles in one or two of those days and not jumping 10 miles six times a week.

This approach also provides positive reinforcement for your targeted "muscles".

The more you set and achieve goals, the more you can set and achieve.

Observing food triggers is another sustainable weight loss solution.

Do you eat when you are bored, stressed or happy? Do you go out with your colleagues every Friday night out of habit? Do you automatically grab a bag of pretzels when you sit down to watch your favorite TV show?

Take a look at your current eating habits and find out what those triggers are, whether positive or negative. Then, systematically try to modify these behaviors based on knowledge of the triggers.

However, this approach to weight loss isn't for everyone, especially with so many ads popping up online for "sexy" weight loss options.

But many people burn out trying the latest diet or cool workout. Eventually people come up to me and say, I'm sick of dieting, I'm sick of yo-yoing, I'm sick of failing. They get to the point where they know there is more to it than food and exercise.

Simple tips for a healthier diet

A diet rich in fruits and vegetables has been scientifically proven to provide many health benefits such as: B. Reduce the risk of several chronic diseases and keep your body healthy.

However, making big changes to your diet can sometimes feel overwhelming.

Instead of making big changes, it might be better to start with a few smaller ones. And it's probably easier to start with one thing than all at once.

Below are small changes that can make regular eating a little healthier. Remember that you don't have to do them all at once. Instead, you may want to add these changes to your life over time.

Slow down

The pace at which you eat affects how much you eat and the likelihood of gaining weight.

In fact, studies comparing different feeding rates show that fast eaters are much more likely to overeat and have a higher body mass index (BMI) than slow eaters. Your appetite, the amount of food you eat, and your satiety are all controlled by hormones. Hormones tell your brain if you are hungry or full.

However, it takes your brain about 20 minutes to receive these messages. That's why eating more slowly can give your brain the time it needs to recognize that you're full.

Studies have backed this up, showing that slow eating can reduce the number of calories you eat at mealtimes and help you lose weight. Eating slowly has also been linked to deeper chewing, which has also been linked to better weight management.

So, just eating slower and chewing more often can help you eat less.

Choose whole meal bread instead of refined bread

You can easily make your diet a little healthier by choosing whole meal bread instead of the traditional refined grain bread.

Refined grains have been linked to many health problems. Whole grains, on the other hand, have been linked to various health benefits, including a reduced risk of type 2 diabetes, heart disease and cancer.

They are also a good source for:

- fiber
- B vitamins
- Minerals like zinc, iron, magnesium and manganese.

There are many varieties of whole wheat bread, and many of them even taste better than refined bread.

Just read the label to make sure your bread is made with only whole grains and not a mix of whole grains and refined grains. It is also best if the bread contains whole seeds or grains.

Add Greek yogurt to your diet

Greek yogurt (or Greek yogurt) is thicker and creamier than regular yogurt.

It is filtered to remove excess whey, the watery part of the milk. This results in a final product that is richer in fat and protein than regular yogurt.

In fact, it contains up to double the protein compared to the same amount of plain yogurt, i.e. up to 10 grams per 100 grams. Eating a good source of protein can help you feel full for longer, which can help control your appetite and reduce your food intake, if that's your goal.

And because Greek yogurt is filtered, it contains fewer carbohydrates and less lactose than regular yogurt. This makes it suitable for people who are on a low-carb diet or are lactose intolerant.

Simply swap a few snacks or regular yogurt varieties with Greek yogurt for a healthy dose of protein and nutrients.

Make sure you choose the plain, unflavored varieties. Flavored yogurt can be packaged with added sugar and other less nutritious ingredients.

Don't shop without a list

There are two main strategies you can use when shopping: make your grocery list in advance and don't go to the store hungry.

Not knowing exactly what you need leaves room for impulse purchases, while hunger can cause you to throw even more low-nutrient foods into the grocery cart.

Therefore, the best strategy is to plan ahead and write down what you need in advance. By doing this and by sticking to your list, you will not only buy healthier items for your home, but you will also save money.

Eat eggs, preferably for breakfast

Eggs are incredibly healthy, especially when eaten in the morning.

They are high in quality protein and many essential nutrients that people often lack, such as choline.

When you look at studies comparing different types of breakfast at equal calories, eggs come out on top.

Eating eggs in the morning increases the feeling of satiety. This has been shown to cause people to consume fewer calories in subsequent meals. Losing weight can be very beneficial if that is your goal.

For example, a study of 50 people found that eating an egg-based breakfast reduced hunger pangs and the amount of calories consumed throughout the day compared to a cereal-based breakfast.

So simply replacing your current breakfast with eggs can already have important health benefits.

Increase your protein intake

Protein is often referred to as the king of nutrients and appears to have some superpowers.

Due to its ability to affect hunger and satiety hormones, it is often considered the richest in macronutrients.

One study found that eating a protein-rich meal lowered levels of the hunger hormone ghrelin more than a carbohydrate-rich meal in obese people.

Additionally, protein helps maintain muscle mass and can even slightly increase the number of calories burned per day. It is also important to avoid the loss of muscle mass that can occur with weight loss and aging. If you're trying to lose weight, try adding a protein source to every meal and snack. This will help you feel full longer, reduce cravings, and reduce the risk of overeating.

Good sources of protein are:

- Dairy products
- Nuts
- Peanut Butter
- Eggs
- Beans
- lean meat

Drink enough water

Drinking enough water is important for your health.

Numerous studies have shown that drinking water can increase weight loss and help maintain weight, and may even slightly increase the number of calories you burn each day. Studies also show that drinking water before meals can reduce appetite and food intake at the next meal.

That said, the important thing is to drink water rather than other drinks. This can dramatically reduce your sugar and calorie intake.

Drinking water regularly can also be associated with better nutritional quality and can reduce the calorie intake of drinks.

Bake or roast instead of grilling or roasting

How you prepare food can drastically change the effects on your health.

Grilling, roasting, roasting and frying are all popular methods of cooking meat and fish.

However, several potentially toxic compounds are formed during these types of cooking methods. Among which:

- polycyclic aromatic hydrocarbons
- advanced glycation end products
- heterocyclic amines

All of these compounds have been linked to a variety of health problems, including cancer and heart disease.

Healthier cooking methods include:

- baking
- roast
- poaching
- pressure cooking
- simmer over low heat
- Slow cooking
- stew
- vacuum packed

These methods do not promote the formation of these harmful compounds and can make food healthier. While you can enjoy a grilled or fried dish from time to time, these methods are best used in moderation.

Take Omega-3 and Vitamin D supplements

About 1 billion people worldwide are vitamin D deficient.

Vitamin D is a fat-soluble vitamin that is very important for bone health and the proper functioning of the immune system. In fact, every cell in your body has a vitamin D receptor, which indicates its importance.

Vitamin D is found in very few foods, but fatty seafood generally contains the highest amounts. Omega-3 fatty acids are another common missing nutrient in fatty seafood. These have many important roles in the body, including reducing inflammation, maintaining heart health, and promoting healthy brain function.

The Western diet is generally very high in omega-6 fatty acids, which increase inflammation and are linked to many chronic diseases. Omega-3 fatty acids help fight this inflammation and keep your body in a more balanced state.

If you don't eat fatty seafood regularly, consider taking a supplement. Omega-3 fatty acids and vitamin D are often found together in many dietary supplements.

Substitute your favorite fast food

Eating out doesn't have to be unhealthy.

Consider upgrading your favorite fast food restaurant to one with healthier options.

There are many healthy fast food restaurants and fusion restaurants that offer healthy and delicious meals. They may just be a great substitute for your favorite burger or pizza. Plus, you can usually get these meals for a very reasonable price.

Try at least one healthy new recipe a week.

Deciding what to eat for dinner can be a constant source of frustration, which is why many people tend to use the same recipes over and over again. Chances are you've been cooking the same recipes on autopilot for years. Whether it's healthy or unhealthy recipes, trying something new can be a fun way to add variety to your diet.

Try to make a healthy new recipe at least once a week. It can change your food and nutrient intake and hopefully add new nutritious recipes to your routine.

You can also try creating a healthier version of a favorite recipe by experimenting with new ingredients, herbs and spices.

Choose hash browns instead of fries

Potatoes are very nutritious and a common accompaniment to many dishes. However, the method of their preparation largely determines their effect on health.

For starters, 3.5 ounces (100 grams) of baked potatoes have 93 calories, while the same amount of fries has more than triple that (333 calories).

Additionally, fried French fries usually contain harmful compounds like aldehydes and trans fats.

Replacing your fries with baked or boiled potatoes is a great way to cut calories and avoid these unhealthy compounds.

Eat your vegetables first

A great way to make sure you eat your vegetables is to enjoy them as an appetizer.

That way, you'll likely finish all your greens when you're hungriest. This can cause you to eat less of other, possibly less healthy parts of the meal later on.

This can cause you to eat fewer and healthier calories, which can lead to weight loss. Eating vegetables before a high-carb meal has also been shown to have positive effects on blood sugar levels.

It slows the rate at which carbohydrates are absorbed into the bloodstream and may benefit short- and long-term blood sugar control in people with diabetes.

Eat your fruit instead of drinking it

Fruits are packed with water, fiber, vitamins and antioxidants.

Studies have repeatedly linked fruit consumption to a reduced risk of various health problems, such as heart disease, type 2 diabetes, and cancer. Since fruits contain fiber and various plant compounds, their natural sugars are generally digested very slowly and do not cause severe blood sugar spikes.

However, the same is not true for fruit juices.

Many fruit juices are not even made of real fruit, but of concentrate and sugar. Some varieties may even contain as much sugar as a sweetened soda.

Even real fruit juices lack the fiber and chewing resistance of whole fruits. This makes fruit juice much more likely to spike your blood sugar, causing you to consume too much in one sitting.

Cook at home more often

Try to make it a habit to cook at home most nights rather than eating out.

First, it's easier for your budget.

Secondly, by cooking the food yourself, you know exactly what is inside. You don't have to worry about hidden unhealthy or high calorie ingredients. If you prepare large portions, you also have leftovers for the next day and even ensure a healthy meal.

Finally, home cooking has been associated with a lower risk of obesity and better diet quality, especially in children.

Be more active

Good nutrition and exercise often go hand in hand. Exercise has been shown to improve your mood and reduce feelings of depression, anxiety and stress. These are the feelings most likely to contribute to emotional eating and binge eating.

In addition to strengthening your muscles and bones, exercise can help you:

- losing weight
- Increase your energy levels
- Reduce your risk of chronic diseases
- improve your sleep

Aim for around 30 minutes of moderate-to-vigorous intensity exercise each day, or just take the stairs and take short walks whenever possible.

Replace sugary drinks with sparkling water

Sugary drinks can be the **unhealthiest** thing you can drink.

They're loaded with added sugars that have been linked to many ailments, including:

- heart disease
- Obesity
- Type 2 diabetes

Also, the sugars in these drinks do not affect the appetite like regular foods do. This means that you don't compensate for the calories you drink by eating less.

A 16-ounce (492 ml) sugary soda contains about 207 calories.

Try replacing your sugary drink with a sugar-free alternative, or simply choose plain or sparkling water instead. This reduces unnecessary calories and reduces excess sugar consumption.

Stay away from "diet" foods

So-called diet foods can be very misleading. They are generally very low in fat and are often labeled "fat free", "low fat", "reduced fat", or "low calorie".

However, to compensate for the loss of flavor and texture due to fat, sugar and other ingredients are often added.

As a result, many diet foods end up containing more sugar and sometimes even more calories than their high-fat counterparts.

Instead, opt for whole foods like fruits and vegetables.

Get a good night's rest

The importance of a good night's sleep cannot be stressed enough.

Sleep deprivation disrupts appetite regulation, often leading to an increase in appetite. This results in increased calorie intake and weight gain.

In fact, people who sleep too little tend to weigh a lot more than people who get enough sleep.

Sleep deprivation also negatively affects concentration, productivity, athletic performance, glucose metabolism, and immune function. Plus, it increases your risk of several diseases, including inflammatory diseases and heart disease.

For this reason, it is important to try to get enough good quality sleep, preferably on a lap.

Eat fresh berries instead of dried ones

Berries are very healthy and full of nutrients, fiber and antioxidants. Most varieties can be purchased fresh, frozen or dried. While all varieties are relatively healthy, dried varieties are a much more concentrated source of calories and sugar as all the water has been removed.

A 100-gram serving of fresh or frozen strawberries contains 31-35 calories, while 100 grams of dried strawberries contain a whopping 375 calories.

Dried varieties are also often coated in sugar, further increasing the sugar content.

By choosing the fresh varieties, you get a much juicier snack that contains less sugar and fewer calories.

Choose popcorn over fries

It may come as a surprise that popcorn is a whole grain loaded with nutrients and fiber.

A 3.5-ounce (100-gram) serving of air-popped popcorn has 387 calories and 15 grams of fiber, while the same amount of potato chips has 532 calories and just 3 grams of fiber.

Consuming whole grains has been linked to health benefits, such as a reduced risk of inflammation and heart disease.

For a healthy snack, try making your own popcorn at home (not microwave popcorn varieties) or buy air-popped popcorn.

Many commercial varieties prepare their popcorn with fat, sugar, and salt, making it no healthier than potato chips.

Choose healthy oils

Highly processed seed and vegetable oils have become a household staple over the past few decades.

Examples include soybean, cottonseed, sunflower and canola oils.

These oils are high in omega-6s but low in heart-healthy omega-3s.

Some research suggests that high ratios of omega-6 to omega-3 can lead to inflammation and have been linked to chronic diseases such as heart disease, cancer, osteoporosis and autoimmune diseases. Replace these oils with healthier alternatives, such as:

- Extra virgin olive oil
- Avocado oil
- Coconut oil

Eat on smaller plates

The size of your dishes has been proven to affect how much you eat.

Eating from a large plate can make your portion appear smaller, while eating from a small plate can make it appear larger.

Eating from a smaller plate was associated with increased feelings of fullness and decreased energy intake in healthy-weight participants.

If you don't eat more than usual, you won't compensate by eating less at the next meal. By eating in smaller dishes, you can trick your brain into thinking you're eating more, making you less likely to overeat.

Put the dressing aside

For many, being able to order a salad in a restaurant is a feat.

However, not all salads are equally healthy. In fact, some salads are topped with high-calorie dressings, which can make the salads even more calorie-dense than other menu items. If you order the dressing on the side, it's much easier to control portion sizes and the amount of calories you eat.

Drink your coffee black

Coffee, one of the most popular drinks in the world, is very healthy.

In fact, it is an important source of antioxidants and has been linked to numerous health benefits such as: B. reduced risk of type 2 diabetes, mental decline and liver disease.

However, many commercial coffees contain many additional ingredients such as sugar, syrup, whipped cream, and sweeteners. Drinking these varieties quickly negates all the health benefits of coffee and instead adds a lot of extra sugar and calories.

Instead, try drinking your coffee black or just add a small amount of milk or cream instead of sugar.

The final result

A complete overhaul of your diet all at once can be a recipe for disaster.

Instead, try incorporating some of the small changes listed above to make your diet healthier.

Some of these tips will help you keep portions reasonable, while others will help you add nutrients or get used to something new. Together they will have a big impact in making your overall diet healthier and more sustainable, without a huge change in your habits.

Most Popular Healthy Thai Dishes

Healthy Eating

It's easy to feel bombarded by the latest health food trends or trendy ingredients. But good nutrition is actually about consistently choosing healthy foods and beverages. With healthy eating habits, it is possible to enjoy foods and beverages that reflect your preferences, cultural traditions and financial considerations.

A healthy diet emphasizes fruits, vegetables, whole grains, dairy products and proteins. Milk recommendations include low-fat or fat-free milk, lactose-free milk, and fortified soy beverages. Other vegetable drinks do not have the same nutritional properties as animal milk and soy drinks. Protein recommendations include seafood, lean meats and poultry, eggs, legumes (beans, peas and lentils), soy products, nuts and seeds.

Most people in the United States need to adjust their eating habits to increase their fiber, calcium, vitamin D, and potassium intake. At the same time, we need to consume less added sugars, saturated fats and sodium. Here are a few ways to get started. bump fiber

Fiber helps maintain digestive health and helps us feel full longer. Fiber also helps control blood sugar and lower cholesterol. Fresh fruits and vegetables, whole grains, legumes, nuts and seeds are good sources of fiber.

To bulk up the fiber, try the following:

• Slice raw vegetables for a quick snack. Storing celery and carrots in water in the refrigerator will keep them crisp longer. • Start your day with a whole grain such as rolled oats or foods containing bulgur or teff. Top your muesli with berries, pumpkin seeds or almonds for even more fiber.

• Add ½ cup of beans or lentils to your salad to add fiber, texture and flavor.

• Enjoy whole fruit, such as a pear, apple, melon wedge or passion fruit, with a meal or as a dessert.

Increase calcium and vitamin D

Calcium and vitamin D work together to support optimal bone health. Our bodies can produce vitamin D from sunlight, but some people may have trouble producing enough vitamin D, and too much sun exposure can increase the risk of skin cancer. Although very few foods naturally contain vitamin D, many foods and beverages are fortified with this essential nutrient.

To increase calcium and vitamin D intake, try the following:

• Drink a fortified milk drink with your meals.

• When preparing your lunch, include a packet of salmon or a can of sardines once a week. Bone-in salmon and sardines contain more calcium than bone-in salmon and sardines. • Add spinach, collard greens, bok choy, mushrooms and taro root to your vegetable dishes.

• Look for foods fortified with calcium and vitamin D. Soy beverages, soy yogurt, orange juice and some whole grains may contain these additional nutrients. Just make sure they don't contain added sugar!

Add more potassium

Potassium helps the kidneys, heart, muscles and nerves to function properly. Too little potassium can raise blood pressure, deplete calcium in bones, and increase the risk of kidney stones. People with chronic kidney disease and those taking certain medications may have too much potassium in their blood. But most people in the United States need more potassium in their diets.

Try this to add more potassium:

• Try new recipes with beets, lima beans or chard.

• Add some variety to your drinks with a cup of 100% prune juice or 100% pomegranate juice.

• Have a banana as a snack. • Enjoy 100% orange juice or a recommended dairy product with meals.

Limit added sugars

Too much added sugar in the diet can contribute to weight gain, obesity, type 2 diabetes, and heart disease. Some foods such as fruit and milk contain natural sugars. Added sugars are sugars and syrups that are added to foods and drinks when they are processed or prepared. Added sugars have many different names, such as cane juice, corn syrup, dextrose, and fructose. Table sugar, maple syrup and honey are also considered added sugars. Sugary drinks are a common source of added sugar

To limit added sugar, try the following:

• Drink water instead of sugary drinks. Add berries or slices of lime, lemon or cucumber for extra flavor.

• Add fruit to your muesli or yogurt to make it sweeter.

- Don't fill up on sugary drinks and snacks. Instead, drink water and have sliced fruits and vegetables on hand for snacks.

- Avoid flavored syrups and whipped cream in cafes. Ask for low-fat or fat-free milk or an unsweetened fortified soy beverage. Or go back to basics with black coffee.

- Read nutrition information and choose foods with little or no added sugar.

Replace saturated fats

Replacing saturated fats with healthier unsaturated fats can help protect your heart. Common sources of saturated fat are fatty meats like ribs and sausages, whole milk, whole cheese, butter, and cream cheese.

We need dietary fat to give us energy, help us develop healthy cells, and help us absorb certain vitamins and minerals. But unsaturated fats are better for us than saturated fats.

To replace saturated fat with unsaturated fat, try the following:

• Replace whole milk in a smoothie with low-fat yogurt and an avocado. • Instead of cheese, sprinkle nuts or seeds on salads.

• Use beans or seafood instead of meat as a source of protein.

• Cook with canola, corn, olive, peanut, safflower, soy or sunflower oil instead of butter or margarine.

• Replace whole milk and cheese with low-fat or fat-free versions.

Avoid sodium

Eating too much sodium can increase your risk of high blood pressure, heart attack, and stroke. More than 70% of the sodium Americans consume comes from packaged and prepared foods. Although sodium comes in many forms, 90% of the sodium we consume comes from salt.

Try this to cut down on sodium:

• Instead of using salt, you can spice up your meals with a squeeze of lemon juice, a pinch of salt-free spice mixes or fresh herbs.

• Eat less processed, prepackaged foods with a high sodium content. Many common foods, including bread, pizza, and processed meats, contain high amounts of sodium. • Check the nutrition label at the grocery store to find products lower in sodium.

• Buy unprocessed foods, such as fresh or frozen vegetables, to prepare at home without salt.

Aim for a variety of colors

A good practice is to aim for a variety of colors on your plate. Fruits and vegetables like dark leafy greens, oranges, and tomatoes — even fresh herbs — are packed with vitamins, fiber, and minerals.

Try that:

• Scatter fresh herbs over salad or whole wheat pasta. • Prepare a red sauce with fresh tomatoes (or low-sodium or no-salt-added canned tomatoes), fresh herbs and spices.

- Add diced vegetables – like peppers, broccoli or onions – to stews and omelettes to add color and nutrition.
- Fill low-fat, unsweetened yogurt with your favorite fruit.

What is the Candida diet?

Candidiasis, commonly known as "Candida", is a fungal infection that can affect men and women of all ages in different parts of the body. It most commonly occurs in the mouth, ears, nose, toenails, fingernails, gastrointestinal tract, and vagina.

Possible symptoms include a veritable laundry list, ranging from bad breath to persistent heartburn to arthritis. Due to its many and varied symptoms, Candida is often overlooked, undiagnosed, or misdiagnosed.

If you have candida or know someone who does, the good news is that there are many natural treatments for candida. The main natural treatment is to change your diet to prevent yeast overgrowth. However, before starting your new diet, it is a good idea to start with a candida cleanse to help the body eliminate excess candida by reddening the digestive tract.

You have two options for a cleanse: a liquid-only cleanse or a milder food cleanse. You can also start with cleaning the first step and then move on to the second step.

Cleaning step 1: Candida cleanse with liquids only (duration 1-2 days)

Start by making a vegetable broth with organic onions, garlic, celery, kale, sea salt, and pure water. Let it simmer and strain. Discard the vegetables and refrigerate the broth.

Drink hot broth throughout the day. Drinking plenty of water is imperative to help your body eliminate all toxins from your system.

While this is not a long-term cleansing, it can be repeated every few weeks as needed. It can also be used as a starting point for cleaning up the underlying food. Cleaning phase 2: steamed vegetables (duration 3-5 days)

Eliminating grains, sugars, fruits, starches, and alcohol from your diet for three to five days can go a long way in your fight against candida overgrowth.

What can you eat on a candida diet? You should especially eat:

• Fresh and organic steamed vegetables. For this cleansing phase, stay away from starchy vegetables like carrots, radishes, beets, sweet potatoes, and white potatoes, which can contribute to high sugar levels and nourish candida.

• Continue to drink plenty of clean water, at least 72 ounces per day, to eliminate candida and its derivatives from your system. • During this period, no more than once a day, you can eat salads based on leafy vegetables (such as Romaine) or bitter vegetables (such as Swiss chard) and garnish with a little coconut oil and apple cider vinegar (or lemon).

During one of the candida cleanses above, you can use bentonite clay to surround toxins and effectively remove them from your system.

Once you are done with the cleansing phase, you can move on to an antifungal diet that not only discourages candida, but helps your body get rid of candida forever!

Here are the dietary steps I recommend for a candida-free diet:

Diet Phase 1:

Eliminate the Food Problem

Now you know what to eat, but you are probably wondering what not to eat on a candida diet. First, you should continue eliminating foods that literally feed candida from your diet and encourage it to thrive in your body.

The biggest offenders include:

- sugar
- White flower
- yeast
- alcohol

These elements are believed to promote candida overgrowth. If you don't eat sugar and white flour, you'll easily eliminate most processed foods, which are generally higher in calories, unhealthy, and low-nutritional ingredients.

Avoiding sugar in all its forms is really the key to fighting candida. Candida yeast cells need sugar to build their cell walls, expand their colonies, and transition to their more virulent fungal form.

That's why a low-sugar diet is such a necessary part of your Candida treatment. If you need help, here's how to beat your sugar addiction.

Going forward, you want your diet to focus on:

• Vegetables

• high quality protein foods

• gluten-free grains (like brown rice and millet)

It is also generally recommended to avoid fruit at this time because, although fruit is very healthy, it is converted into sugar in the body. In terms of vegetables, you should also avoid these slightly sweet and starchy varieties:

• potatoes

• roots

• sweet potatoes

• Sweet potato

• beets

• peas

• parsnip

These veggies have been banned from a strict anti-candida diet due to their high carbohydrate content, but they are definitely nutritious and can be reintroduced later in the treatment.

Diet Step 2:

Increase your Candida Killers intake and boost your immune system

You want to make sure you include items from my top 10 list below on a daily basis, including:

1. apple cider vinegar
2. green vegetables
3. green drinks
4. coconut oil
5. Manuka honey
6. garlic
7. ground chia and flax seeds
8. Unsweetened cranberry juice
9. cultured dairy products

10. Spices (like turmeric and cinnamon)

How long do I have to eat like this?

It takes a few weeks to several months to be successful on the Candida diet. It really depends on the person and a few key variables:

• how strict you are on this diet

• the intake and effectiveness of probiotics and antifungals

• the severity of your candida

Step 3 of the diet:

Reintroduce Forbidden Foods

Once you are free of your symptoms of candida and candida itself, what then? As you might have guessed, going back to your old habits and eating habits will likely only bring candida back. However, you can gradually reintroduce certain foods into your new Candida diet.

Low-sugar fruits like green apples are a good example of a smart choice. If the foods you're reintroducing aren't causing Candida symptom flare-ups, you can move on to reintroducing other foods you've been avoiding.

I recommend doing this reintroduction slowly and step by step.

best foods

Here are some of the foods to eat while on the candida diet.

1. Apple cider vinegar

The acid and enzymes in apple cider vinegar have been shown to help kill and eliminate excess yeast in the body.

2. Green vegetables and green drinks

Leafy green vegetables help alkalize the body by fighting the acidic nature of yeast overgrowth. Research suggests that green vegetables are sugar-free, but contain high amounts of magnesium, which naturally detoxifies the body, vitamin C to boost the immune system, chlorophyll to cleanse the body, B vitamins to fuel body and iron for full support. from the body. 3. Coconut oil

Coconut oil has antimicrobial properties and studies show that the combination of lauric acid and caprylic acid found in coconut oil kills harmful candida when ingested and applied topically.

4. Stevia

We know that sugar feeds candida. For this reason, it's important to use a variety of sweeteners, and stevia is a perfect choice for those on a candida diet. Studies show that stevia is not only an antifungal, anti-inflammatory, and antibiotic, but also helps balance the pancreas, which is often compromised when a person has candida.

5. Garlic

Garlic contains a large number of sulfur compounds which have extremely potent broad-spectrum antifungal properties. Animal studies conclude that raw garlic is particularly effective in the fight against Candida.

6. Ground flax seeds and chia seeds

The polyphenols in flax seeds and chia seeds have been found to support the growth of probiotics in the gut and may also help eliminate yeast and candida in the body.

7. Unsweetened cranberry juice

Cranberry juice with no added sugar has been shown to help correct the pH level of urine, preventing the overgrowth of fungi such as candida.

8. Kefir

Goat's milk kefir has shown antibacterial and anti-candida effects in animal studies.

9. Spices like turmeric and cinnamon

Turmeric contains an active ingredient called curcumin which completely inhibits the growth of Candida albicans (as well as many other fungal strains). Cinnamon can treat oral thrush because studies have shown that people who take cinnamon supplements are generally less likely to suffer from Candida overgrowth than those who don't.

10. Boiled vegetables

Cooked, non-starchy vegetables — like broccoli, cauliflower, and asparagus — provide valuable candida-fighting nutrients.

11. Organic meat

Proteins play a key role in Candida. If you get your protein from factory-raised meat, you might actually be feeding Candida, while research suggests that foods high in healthy fats and protein protect against Candida. This is why it is so important to consume only organic and farm-raised meat.

12. bone broth

Bone broth benefits many different aspects of our health, and you can add candida treatment to the list. In fact, it's one of the best food sources for destroying candida due to its positive effects on gut health.

13. Pau D'Arco Tea

Pau d'Arco tea is probably the #1 thing to add to your candida diet. It helps the body fight Candida naturally. This is because it is proven to contain antifungal compounds like lapachol, which have been proven to fight candida.

Avoid Foods

Here are the foods to avoid on the candida diet.

1. Sugar and sugar substitutes

These sweet things feed yeast, so avoid them at all costs.

2. fruits and fruit juices

Although fruits are generally healthy, they are high in sugar and can make candidiasis worse.

3. Alcohol

Most alcohols contain yeast, so it's no surprise that more of it is produced when consumed. It should be avoided.

4. cereals

Grains break down into sugar and can feed candida, yeast, and bad bacteria.

5. Vinegar

All types of vinegar should be avoided for candida overgrowth, with the exception of apple cider vinegar. Apple cider vinegar is the only vinegar that alkalizes the body and kills candida.

6. peanuts

Peanuts can often contain mold, which only promotes the growth of candida. Additionally, peanut allergy is one of the most common food allergies in the world, which is another reason to avoid peanuts.

7. Dairy products

Unless it's fermented, you'll want to avoid dairy products in the early stages of your cleanup. Milk contains lactose, which is a sugar.

8. Food intolerances

Some yeast infections are caused by food allergies. Try to avoid foods that cause negative reactions of any kind.

If you think you have a food allergy or sensitivity, try an elimination diet to find out which foods are causing the intolerance.

Other foods to avoid are:

- Dried fruit
- Bananas
- Frozen drinks

Essential Oils for Candida

Some of the best oils for fighting Candida are:

- Oil of oregano
- Myrrh oil
- Lavender oil
- Clove oil

These help kill a variety of parasites and fungi, including Candida, in the body. Lavender oil has been shown to inhibit the growth of

Candida and is effective in preventing the infection from spreading.

By mixing a few drops of clove oil or lavender oil with coconut oil during your cleanse, you can help kill the offending candida. However, since these essential oils are powerful, they should only be taken internally for 10 days or less.

For oral thrush, you can use three drops of clove oil with a tablespoon of coconut oil and swirl the mixture in your mouth for 20 minutes. This oil pulling is great for killing candida and general body detox. The best supplements

These supplements can help with your candida diet:

1. Probiotics (50 billion units per day)

Give your body healthy bacteria, which can help reduce the presence of yeast.

2. Oregano oil (2 drops 3 times a day for 7 days and then stop)

Oregano oil is naturally antibacterial and antifungal.

3. Garlic (2 caps or cloves per day)

Helps fight fungal infections and strengthen the immune system.

4. Vitamin C (1,000 milligrams, 2-3 times a day)

It strengthens the immune function and helps fight infections.

5. Grapefruit Seed Extract (200 milligrams, 2-3 times a day)

Pure grapefruit seed extract can kill a variety of infectious microbes and even help fight common health problems like candida and athlete's foot. 6. Turkey Tail Mushroom (1 gram, 2-3 times a day)

Also known as Trametes versicolor, research published in Frontiers in Microbiology shows that turkey tail's antimicrobial activities can help treat candida. Additionally, the prebiotics in turkey tail help the microbiome and help food bacteria grow, improving overall gut health.

7. Astragalus root (1 gram, 2-3 times a day)

Another good supplement for healthy gut flora, animal research shows how astragalus can alter the gut microbiota and increase beneficial bacteria. Therefore, it can fight candida and other fungi while maintaining a healthy microbiome.

Additionally, you can use the following herbs to treat candida:

- olive leaf
- other mushrooms

A 2003 in vitro study conducted by Israel showed that olive leaf extracts have an antimicrobial effect against bacteria and fungi. Olive leaf extracts killed almost all bacteria tested, including dermatophytes (which cause infections on the skin, hair and nails), candida albicans (a causative agent of oral and genital infections) and Escherichia coli (bacteria in the lower intestine).

Meal times and recipes

You definitely want to eat a mix of raw and cooked vegetables on the candida diet. The idea is to eliminate foods compatible with candida while expelling those that promote candida growth. Here's an example tag to get you started:

• Breakfast: egg and vegetable omelette with broccoli, onions, salt and pepper

• Snack: trail mix with almonds, walnuts and macadamia nuts

• Lunch: Grilled chicken on salad with spinach, slivered almonds, avocado and lemon vinaigrette

• Snack: A cup of real bone broth or green tea

• Dinner: wild salmon fillet seasoned with cilantro and topped with a bed of kale and olive oil vinaigrette

• Dessert: piece of high quality dark chocolate

When it comes to recipes, you obviously want ones that omit all of the candida-boosting foods listed above, while including as many candida killers as possible.

• This Green Detox Machine juice recipe is a great addition to any Candida diet.

• Containing steak, leafy greens and quality vegetables, this Buddha Bowl is a great option once you've started reintroducing a variety of vegetables into your diet.

• This salmon coleslaw is made with fresh salmon fillet and a simple lemon vinaigrette.

Precautions: Candida Death Symptoms

Quickly killing the candida in your body triggers a metabolic reaction that releases over 70 different toxins into your body. Sounds pretty intense, right?

Before being put off, what you may or may not have to deal with as a result of candida death is definitely preferable to what you will face if you let the candida bloom internally.

Symptoms that show candida cleansing and candida diet are working include:

• Decreased brain function

• Headache

• Fatigue

• Dizziness

- Bowel problems, including bloating, gas, constipation and nausea
- Sweating and fever
- Sinusitis
- Skin pimples (not limited to the face)
- Typical flu-like symptoms. These symptoms usually disappear within 7-10 days. The candida leaves your body, and within a few weeks, you will notice an increase in energy and focus, as well as relief from other symptoms you have been experiencing. If you are experiencing chronic or unusually persistent candida infections, you should see your doctor. This could be a sign of an underlying disease, such as diabetes or a dysfunction of the immune system, which creates a more favorable environment for candida to grow.

Final thoughts

- Candida is unfortunately a common problem for many people. Symptoms are often ignored, undiagnosed, or misdiagnosed.
- An antifungal diet can reduce and eliminate candida and its unpleasant symptoms. Some

of the dietary changes may need to be long-term if reintroducing certain foods is not successful.

• Your improved health and energy levels are worth any food or drink you miss.

• In general, it's always best to avoid sugary and processed foods for your overall health. Real, whole, living foods are always the best choice!

This content is for informational and educational purposes only. It is not intended to provide medical advice or to replace such advice or treatment from a personal physician. All readers / viewers of this content are advised to consult their physician or qualified healthcare professionals for specific health issues. Neither Dr. Neither Ax nor the publisher of this content are responsible for any health consequences of any person or persons who read or follow the information contained in this educational content. All viewers of this content, especially those taking prescription or over-the-counter medications, should consult with their physician before embarking on any nutrition, supplement, or lifestyle program.

The Candida Diet: Top Five Foods to Eat and Avoid

So far in this section, we have looked at the causes and symptoms of Candida overgrowth (or yeast infection).

In this section, we'll take a look at what you can and can't eat when dealing with Candida overgrowth. I'll give you the most common foods that feed Candida and contribute to symptoms and the best foods you can eat to suppress and control it.

As we've seen in this series, Candida is a simple organism that doesn't take long to thrive. The moist, warm environment of our digestive system, a reduction in healthy bacteria (usually caused by taking antibiotics), and lots of sugar are all it takes for Candida to grow, thrive, and become established in your gut, causing a host of discomfort symptoms such as indigestion causing symptoms, emotional problems, skin problems, weight problems, muscle and joint pain, food allergies, itching and frequent infections for n to name a few. These symptoms alone and in combination all contribute to making you feel seriously below average. However, a few simple changes to your diet can help alleviate them all. Isn't that great news?

If you have or suspect you have candida, there are steps you can take to minimize candida growth, starting with your diet. Here is a list of foods that I have found to be the worst for people with candida overgrowth in my naturopathic practice.

The five most important foods to avoid

1. Sugar

Any form of processed sugar, including white or brown sugar derived from cane sugar and any simple sweetener derived from maple syrup, honey, agave, brown rice syrup or malt. You should also be very careful to avoid high fructose corn syrup - this processed form of sugar, derived from the corn plant, is particularly problematic for yeast overgrowth and should be eliminated. Read the labels, you might be surprised to find all the hidden sources of sugar you might be consuming. Packaged soups, coffee creams, packaged spices are all potential sources.

2. Simple carbohydrates

Processed carbohydrates such as white flour, white rice contains no fiber and are converted to simple sugars in the digestive system. Foods in this category include crackers, chips, pasta, and noodles.

3. Yeast

Candida is a yeast, and when you consume foods that contain yeast, you add more yeast to an already heavy environment. Foods high in yeast include:

* Alcohol fermented with yeast. Wine and beer contain most of the yeast, and people sensitive to yeast tend to react more to it than to spirits like vodka, gin and tequila, which contain less of it.

* Fermented products including all types of vinegar, soy sauce, tamari, salad dressings, mayonnaise, ketchup, mustard and most other spices containing vinegar.

* Many loaves contain yeast: it is what makes the bread rise, making it airy and light. Sourdough bread gets mixed reviews about being allowed on a Candida diet. Sourdough is made with sourdough, so no active yeast is added to the mix. However, sourdough comes from naturally occurring yeast spores floating around in the environment. For this reason, I recommend avoiding sourdough when doing a candida cleanse. The tortillas do not contain yeast and can be used as a bread substitute.

4. Mold
Foods high in mold can contribute to fungal spores in the intestinal tract which contribute to the growth of Candida. Foods that may have mold include:

* Wrapped, smoked, or cured meats such as hot dogs, smoked salmon, and salt pork bacon.
*Cheeses, especially "mold" cheeses such as Brie and Camembert. I recommend avoiding all cheeses during the candida cleanse.
*Peanuts & Pistachios

* Dried fruit and bottled, canned or jarred fruit. These belong to both the sugar category and the mushroom category, because they contain both concentrated sugar and often also fungal spores on the skin.

5. Mushrooms

Fungi are a fungus and as such can also contribute to yeast overgrowth. Mushrooms play a role in medicine, and some varieties can strengthen the immune system. However, for the purpose of treating Candida, it is best to avoid all foods that contain a fungal component to minimize yeast growth in the gut. The five best foods to eliminate Candida

The best diet to minimize Candida overgrowth is a diet rich in healthy proteins, fats, and complex carbohydrates. Here are my top five food groups to beat Candida:

1. Proteins

Proteins of animal origin such as chicken, fish, shellfish, eggs

Protein from non-animal sources such as beans, legumes (such as red or brown lentils), nuts and seeds (except peanuts and pistachios)

2. Fresh vegetables

Especially dark leafy vegetables like spinach, kale, kale and cabbage. Root vegetables such as carrots and potatoes can be eaten in moderation, but be careful, as they contain carbohydrates that turn into sugar after eating. Frozen, tinned or tinned vegetables can be eaten, but should be eaten in moderation - in general, fresh vegetables are always better.

3. Fresh fruit

1-2 servings of fresh fruit daily provide good fiber, vitamins and minerals. However, if you experience symptoms of bloating, bloating, and brain fog after eating fruit, you may be sensitive to it and should eliminate it from your diet as well.

4. Complex carbohydrates

Some people can manage whole grains in their diet. If you find that you have bloating, bloating, stomach pain, blood sugar crashes, or weight issues after eating whole grains, you should avoid them. Alternatively, you may be able to consume grains such as:

*Oats

*Barley

* Kamut

*Brown or wild rice

*Millet

*Teff

*Buckwheat

*Andean millet

5. Quality oils (good fats)

All of our cells have an outer layer of fat that forms the cell membrane. When we eat high quality oils, this membrane is healthier and functions optimally. When our cell membranes are functioning properly, we are healthier and have more energy. Unrefined, cold-pressed oils are best when available. Good fats include (but are not limited to):

- Coconut oil
- Olive oil (avoid the olives themselves as they are pickled in brine, so they fall into the category of fermented foods and should be avoided)
- Avocados and avocado oil
- Sunflower oil
- Safflower oil
- Fish oil
- Linseed oil
- Chia seeds

In addition to a good diet, it is important to drink enough fluids. Drinking 1-2 liters of water daily contributes to a healthy digestive system and helps minimize yeast overgrowth.

Final Thoughts

Candida overgrowth can be the hidden culprit of many chronic health conditions. It can build up over a long period of time, and symptoms may not be noticeable at first. In my experience, most people would do well to do a Candida cleanse at some point in their life and eliminate sugars and yeast-increasing foods from their diets for a certain period of time. Cleaning up the diet, adding high-quality probiotics, and cutting down on sugar will always help put people on the path to good health.

If you suspect that you have Candida overgrowth and would like to learn more about my specially designed Candida yeast detox program, make an appointment today. It is a three-level assisted treatment that:

- Eliminate food that causes yeast to grow
- Kills yeast
- Repopulate the intestines with healthy bacteria

This concludes the series on Candida overgrowth and its role in your health. Look for my new upcoming book series on deadly food allergies.

www.ingramcontent.com/pod-product-compliance
Lightning Source LLC
LaVergne TN
LVHW050316160826
845677LV00014B/3431
9798848824797